TRACHEOSTOMY RECOVERY RECIPES

Complete Guide Unlocking The Secrets Of Nutrition To Rapid Healing After Surgery Success, Nourishing Meal Plans, Recipes, Tips For Optimal Health Wellness

DR. ALLAN FREDA

Contents

There is a lot of useful information in the book, including healing foods that are designed to help people recover from tracheostomy surgery.

These recipes are meant to give you important nutrients, help your body heal, and improve your general health. Additionally, the book includes flexible meal plans that can help people make food plans that fit their wants and tastes.

In addition, "Tracheostomy Recovery Recipes" includes tips from medical workers to help readers on their way to recovery. These tips cover many areas of post-surgery care, such as what to eat, how to change your lifestyle, and how to stay healthy in the long run.

Overall, this book is a must-have for anyone dealing with the difficulties of tracheostomy healing. It includes useful tips, healthy recipes, and expert opinions to help readers reach their health and wellness goals.

Disclaimer

The information in this book is for informational purposes only and should not replace professional medical advice, diagnosis, or treatment. Always consult your physician or a qualified health provider regarding any medical concerns. Do not disregard professional medical advice or delay seeking it based on information in this book.

The author does not endorse or have affiliations with any mentioned entities. References are for informational purposes only.

Consult your healthcare provider before making dietary or lifestyle changes, especially during recovery from surgery, as individual needs vary.

Results may vary, and the information provided is not guaranteed to produce specific outcomes.

By reading this book, you acknowledge and agree to consult your healthcare provider before implementing any information herein.

For further guidance, consult your healthcare provider or reputable medical websites for reliable information on surgery recovery diets.

CHAPTER 1
AN INTRODUCTION TO RECIPES FOR TRACHEOSTOMY RECOVERY

Surgery called tracheostomy, which involves making a hole in the neck so that the person can breathe, is often needed because of serious breathing problems, injuries, or long-term intubation. While the surgery itself is important for managing breathing, the time it takes to heal after a tracheostomy is just as important.

It involves a multifaceted method that includes medical care, rehabilitation, and, most importantly, food choices. Getting better after having a tracheostomy can be hard because you may have to deal with complications and get used to a new way of life. This guide goes into great detail about the importance of diet in tracheostomy recovery and also looks at a wide range of tracheostomy recovery recipes.

People who have had a tracheostomy can start on the path to better healing, better health, and long-term wellness by learning how these foods work and how they can help with their post-surgery diet.

How to Understand Tracheostomy Recovery

Tracheostomy healing is made up of several stages, and each one has its challenges and needs. At first, care given right after surgery focuses on making sure the airways are open, the wounds are healing, and breathing is stable.

This stage usually takes place in a hospital or intensive care unit, where medical workers are watching over the person. After the acute phase, people move on to the subacute phase, where they continue to heal their wounds, get used to having a tracheostomy tube in their throat, and slowly stop using mechanical breathing. Lastly, the long-term part includes recovery, getting back to normal daily life, and getting used to living with a tracheostomy. During these stages, good nutrition is very important for helping the body recover, boost immune function, repair tissues, and stay healthy generally.

When recovering from a tracheostomy, nutrition is even more important for several reasons. First, people who have a tracheostomy may have trouble eating, which is called dysphagia. This can make it hard for them to eat by mouth and make them more likely to become malnourished.

Having a tracheostomy tube also changes the usual physical and anatomical processes that help with swallowing and protecting the airway, which raises the risk of aspiration and pulmonary complications. So, making sure you get enough food is very important to avoid nutritional deficits, help tissues heal, and lower the risk of complications.

Also, a good diet can boost the immune system, help wounds heal, and build up the muscles in your lungs, all of which speed up recovery and make things better overall. Because of this, a customized, nutrient-dense diet is necessary to meet the specific needs and problems of people who have had a tracheostomy.

Why these recipes can help

Tracheostomy recovery recipes are very helpful for people who need to meet their nutritional needs and dietary limits after having a tracheostomy. These recipes were carefully made to address specific issues like trouble swallowing, the risk of aspiration, and changes in taste perception that are common during tracheostomy healing.

These recipes use flavor-boosting techniques, soft textures, and nutrient-dense ingredients to help people on their way to healing by giving them food, fun, and therapeutic benefits. Tracheostomy recovery recipes also include useful tips for planning meals, making them, and adapting to changes in diet. This gives patients and their caretakers the power to make smart decisions and create a helpful environment that helps people heal. These recipes offer a complete approach to nutrition that is specifically designed for tracheostomy patients. They let you try out new pureed recipes, change the taste of foods, or add immune-boosting ingredients. In the end, tracheostomy recovery recipes are an important part of making sure that people have the best diet possible after surgery, speeding up recovery, and promoting long-term health for people who are dealing with the difficulties of life after tracheostomy.

CHAPTER 2
WHAT YOU NEED AND HOW TO USE IT IN THE KITCHEN

When it comes to recovering from a tracheostomy, nutrition is very important for speeding up the healing process, boosting the immune system, and ensuring general health. It becomes very important to make meals that are not only healthy but also tasty and easy to eat. Let's look at the most important items and kitchen tools you'll need to make this journey a success.

A Look at the Essential Ingredients

When making meals for someone recovering from a tracheostomy, it's important to choose foods that are soft, easy to swallow, and full of nutrients. A well-rounded diet that meets the body's essential needs includes a wide range of foods. Here are some important things to think about:

1. Soft Proteins: Eating soft, lean proteins like eggs, tofu, fish, and ground meats helps your body get enough of the important amino acids it needs to repair tissues and build muscle.

2. Vegetables That Are High in Nutrients: Cooking vegetables until soft or pureeing them gives you the vitamins, minerals, and enzymes your body needs to stay healthy and strong. Spinach, carrots, sweet potatoes, and bananas are some examples.

3. Healthy Fats: Eating foods with healthy fats, like olive oil, avocado oil, nuts, and seeds, helps your body absorb nutrients and gives you energy while you're healing.

4. Full Grains: Muesli, quinoa and brown rice are all soft full grains that are high in fiber, which is good for your digestive health. They also release energy slowly, which makes you feel full and improves your general health.

5. Water: This isn't an ingredient, but staying hydrated is very important for healing. Drink a lot

of water, herbal teas, and clear broths to keep from getting dehydrated and to help your body heal.

A Guide to Kitchen Tools and Equipment

Having the right tools in your kitchen makes it easier to make meals and keeps you safe and comfortable, especially while you're recovering from a tracheostomy. Here is a list of the most important kitchen tools:

1. A blender or food processor is a must-have for making smooth purees and soups from a wide range of ingredients. This makes it easier to eat healthy meals without giving up taste or texture.

2. Strainer or Sieve: A fine-mesh strainer or sieve is useful for getting rid of any lumps or woody bits in pureed foods so that the consistency is smooth and easy to digest.

3. Soft Food Moulds: If you buy silicone molds or ice cube trays, you can divide soft foods into serving sizes and freeze them.

When you're ready to eat them, just thaw them out.

4. Flexible Spatulas and Utensils: Choose spatulas and utensils that are soft and flexible. These will be easier on sensitive mouths and won't hurt or bother them while you're feeding or preparing meals.

5. Electric Steamer or Slow Cooker: These tools make cooking easier by slowly steaming or simmering food, which keeps the nutrients and flavors intact without needing to be watched all the time.

Advice on How to Make Meals

Making meals quickly is important to make sure that you always have healthy foods while you are recovering from a tracheostomy. Here are some ways to speed up the process:

1. Batch cooking: Make a lot of soups, purees, and soft foods ahead of time and divide them into

serving sizes that make them easy to store and reheat during the week.

2. Label and Date: Make sure that each batch of ready-made meals is properly labeled and dated to keep them fresh and safe. For long-term keeping, use containers or bags that can go in the freezer.

3. Texture Modification: Try out different textures and levels of firmness to suit different tastes and swallowing skills. You can change how thick soups and purees are to make them more or less comforting.

4. Flavour Enhancement: To make meals more interesting and varied, add herbs, spices, and sauces to soft foods to make them taste better. To cut down on sodium, don't use too much salt and choose natural spices instead.

5. Health and Safety: Be sure to follow strict cleanliness rules when making meals to keep them from getting contaminated and to lower the risk of

getting an infection, especially for people whose immune systems aren't working well.

knowing the value of key ingredients and having the right kitchen tools are important steps in making the most of your post-surgery diet for tracheostomy recovery. By eating foods that are high in nutrients, using the right kitchen tools, and following best practices when making meals, you can help the body heal, improve your general health, and make sure that your recovery lasts.

CHAPTER 3
SOUPS AND BREAD THAT ARE HIGH IN NUTRIENTS

Tracheostomy recovery can be hard, and you need to look at your whole health to help your body heal and be healthy generally.

Adopting a nutrient-rich diet that helps the body heal and makes the patient stronger and more energetic is an important part of this recovery process.

Soups and broths that are high in nutrients stand out as especially good for you because they are easy to eat, have a lot of health benefits, and can help you feel better.

This part goes into more detail about nutrient-rich soups and broths, talking about how they can help with tracheostomy recovery and giving some healing recipes that can help patients on their way to recovery.

One of the most important parts of a healthy diet after surgery is vegetable broth, which is full of vitamins, minerals, and enzymes that help the body heal. You can make this healing potion with a wide range of veggies, including celery, onions, carrots, and leafy greens. Each one adds a different set of nutrients to the broth.

Carrots, which are high in beta-carotene, give you vitamin A, which is important for your immune system and tissue repair. Celery, on the other hand, gives you flavor and potassium, which is an electrolyte that is important for keeping your fluid balance and muscles working.

As well as adding flavour to the soup, onions contain quercetin, a flavonoid that may help fight cancer and is known to reduce inflammation. Leafy greens, like spinach or kale, give you vitamin

K, which is important for bone health and blood clotting. By simmering these veggies in water or low-sodium vegetable broth, you can get their nutrients out. The result is a tasty and healing drink that you can drink on its own or use as a base for other dishes.

People don't always realize how healthy potatoes are, but they are the star of this creamy and warming soup made especially for people recovering from tracheostomy. Although potatoes don't look very healthy, they are very healthy for you because they are full of vitamin C, potassium, and fiber.

These nutrients are very important for gut health, supporting immune function, and keeping blood pressure in check, all of which are important parts of the healing process. To make this healthy soup, potatoes are peeled, cut into chunks, and cooked until they are soft.

The soup is then blended until it is smooth and velvety. Adding things like low-fat milk or unsweetened almond milk makes it creamier without adding extra calories or saturated fat, so it's good for people who are watching what they eat or who want a lighter choice.

Also, spices like garlic, thyme, or parsley can be added to make the food taste better and give it extra health benefits, like killing germs or reducing inflammation. For those who are recovering from a tracheostomy, this creamy potato soup is a healthy and comforting addition to their diet. It provides nutrition and culinary pleasure.

Chicken bone broth that is good for you:

When it comes to healing from a tracheostomy, chicken bone soup is a nutritional powerhouse. It is loved for having a lot of important nutrients, collagen, and amino acids. In traditional chicken broth, meat and veggies are simmered together.

To make bone broth, bones, usually chicken or beef, are cooked for a long time to get their nutrient-rich marrow and gelatin out. By cooking slowly, you can make a powerful elixir that is full of healing compounds like glucosamine, chondroitin, and gelatin.

These compounds help keep joints healthy, handle food better, and make skin more elastic. Another thing that bone broth does is contain amino acids like glycine and proline, which help the body heal after surgery by reducing inflammation and boosting the immune system.

 When added to a tracheostomy recovery diet, chicken bone broth provides a source of protein that is easy to digest and important minerals.

This helps the body rebuild tissues that were damaged during surgery and replenish nutrient stores. As a warm drink or as a base for soups and stews, chicken bone broth is an important part of a good diet after surgery because it helps the body heal from the inside out.

This warm and healthy soup is made with lentils, which are known for being high in nutrients and useful in many ways. It is designed to help people who have had a tracheostomy recover. Lentils are a complete food that is full of nutrients that are good for you and help you heal.

They contain protein, fiber, complex carbohydrates, and many vitamins and minerals. Their high fiber content is good for your digestive system and keeps your blood sugar levels in check.

The protein in them helps repair tissues and muscles. Also, lentils have a lot of folate, iron, and magnesium, which are important nutrients for making red blood cells, moving oxygen around the body, and using energy.

All of these are important parts of the healing process.

To make this hearty soup, fragrant veggies like onions, garlic, and carrots are simmered with lentils. Herbs and spices like cumin, turmeric, and smoked paprika are also added.

Adding tomatoes or tomato paste to the soup gives it a slight sweetness and sourness. It also gives it lycopene, a powerful antioxidant that may help reduce inflammation. Comforting lentil soup is a hearty meal that can be eaten on its own or with whole grains for extra nutrition. It is a good choice for people who are going through the tough times of tracheostomy healing.

Soups and broths that are high in nutrients are very important for helping people recover from tracheostomy surgery because they provide important nutrients, keep you hydrated, and provide warmth and nourishment while you heal. These recipes are made to meet the specific nutritional needs of people recovering from tracheostomy.

They range from healing veggie broth that is full of vitamins and antioxidants to comforting and filling potato soup. By adding these healing elixirs to their diet, patients can get the best nutrition after surgery, help their tissues heal, and improve their general health for long-term recovery and wellness.

CHAPTER 4
DISHES THAT ARE SOFT AND EASY TO SWALLOW

When recovering from a tracheostomy, nutrition is very important for speeding up the healing process, building strength, and making sure of general health. During this stage, soft, easy-to-swallow foods are very important because they provide nutrition while minimizing pain and other problems that can come up with eating problems. The idea behind this part is to help the healing process by adding soft and gentle recipes to the diet after surgery.

Dishes that are soft and easy to swallow

People who have had tracheostomy surgery often have short or permanent problems swallowing. Because of this, they need to eat foods that are soft and easy to handle. These foods are made to be easy on the throat so that they cause less irritation or pain while still giving you the nutrients you need to heal and get better. People who are recovering from a tracheostomy can keep eating well without making their situation worse by focusing on soft textures and easy-to-swallow consistencies.

People who are recovering from a tracheostomy can eat tender and delicious braised chicken. Once you start cooking the chicken slowly in a liquid like broth or sauce, the meat gets soft and easy to chew. Additionally, braising adds moisture to the chicken, keeping it from drying out or getting tough, which is very important for people who have trouble eating. Seasonings can be changed to suit different tastes and dietary needs, making sure that the food is both tasty and healthy.

People who are recovering from a tracheostomy can eat mashed sweet potatoes as a healthy and comfortable side dish.

When cooked, sweet potatoes are naturally soft, and they're easy to mash into a smooth texture, which makes them great for people who have trouble eating.

 It tastes better with a little honey added to it, and the slight sweetness is nice on the tongue. Besides being tasty, sweet potatoes are also full of fiber, vitamins, and minerals that are good for your health and can help you recover.

Soft eggs steamed with spinach

You can get a lot of protein from soft cooked eggs, which are also easy on the throat and swallow.

By cooking the eggs slowly over low heat and adding things like milk or cream, you can make the texture smoother and softer.

Adding spinach not only makes the dish healthier, but it also gives you extra vitamins and minerals that your body needs to heal and recover.

Soft scrambled eggs with spinach are a great food for people who are healing from tracheostomy surgery because they are high in protein and nutrients.

Smoothies with gentle fruit

Fruit drinks are a flexible and easy way for people recovering from tracheostomy to get important nutrients into their diet. Smoothies are smooth and easy to drink because they are made by mixing soft fruits like bananas, berries, and mangoes with yogurt or milk. You can add spinach, avocado, or protein powder to the drink to make it healthier and raise its nutritional value.

Furthermore, smoothies can be changed to fit specific dietary needs and restrictions, which means they are good for a wide range of people at different points of recovery.

It is important to eat soft, easy-to-swallow foods after surgery to help the body heal and get the best nutrition during tracheostomy rehab.

 By focusing on soft textures and nutrient-dense foods, people who have trouble swallowing can get the nutrition they need while minimizing the pain and problems that come with it.

These recipes not only give you the nutrients you need, but they also make you feel good and help your health and healing last.

CHAPTER 5
TASTY PURÉES AND MIXED MEALS

Tracheostomy is surgery that makes an opening in the windpipe. People who have trouble breathing often need this treatment. During the healing process after a tracheostomy, it is important to pay extra attention to nutrition because the body needs enough food to heal properly.

To avoid problems and speed up healing, it's important to eat soft, easily digestible foods during this time. There are many food choices out there, but delicious purees and blended meals stand out because they are not only tasty but also full of nutrients that are important for healing and maintaining health.

People who are trying to get better from a tracheostomy should eat flavorful purees and blended foods.

These recipes have a smooth feel that is easy on the throat. This makes it easier to swallow and lowers the chance of pain or irritation. They can also be changed to fit specific dietary needs and tastes, making sure that patients get enough food during this important part of their recovery.

Butternut squash is great for tracheostomy healing recipes because it has a great flavor and is full of nutrients. This vegetable can be used in many ways. It is easy to stomach and full of vitamins and minerals that help the immune system work and heal tissues.

To make a smooth butternut squash puree, all you have to do is roast or steam the squash until it's soft and then mix it. Adding a bit of warmth with cinnamon or nutmeg can make the flavor better, making it a comforting and satisfying choice for people who are going through the hard times of recovering from a tracheostomy.

Avocado is known for having a creamy texture and a lot of nutrients. It goes well with yogurt to make a smooth and healthy mix that is great for tracheostomy healing.

Avocados have a lot of vitamins, minerals, and heart-healthy fats. Yoghurt has probiotics that help your gut stay healthy and your immune system work well.

Putting these things in a blender makes a silky-smooth mixture that you can drink by itself or add a little honey or citrus for extra sweetness and tang.

This mix of avocado and yogurt not only gives you important nutrients, but it's also a tasty and refreshing treat for people who want to change up their diet after surgery.

This tracheostomy recovery meal is all about spinach, which is known for being very healthy. Ricotta cheese adds a rich, creamy texture to the dish. Spinach is full of minerals, vitamins, and antioxidants that help the body heal and protect itself. Ricotta adds protein and a smooth taste to the mix.

The spinach needs to be wilted, and then it needs to be blended with ricotta cheese until it is smooth and uniform. The result is a smooth spinach and ricotta mixture that not only tastes great but also gives you a lot of nutrients that you need to help your body heal and stay healthy after a tracheostomy.

Berries, which are loved for their bright colors and antioxidants, can help people who are recovering from a tracheostomy stay cool and healthy.

These little fruits—strawberries, blueberries, raspberries, and blackberries—are very high in vitamins, minerals, and phytonutrients that help the body heal and stay healthy.

To make a mixed berry puree, just blend your favorite berries until they are smooth. If you want a thicker puree, you can add a splash of juice or yogurt. This colorful and tasty stew is not only full of good nutrients, but it also tastes great, which makes it a great addition to a diet after surgery.

tasty purees and blended foods are an important part of the tracheostomy recovery diet because they are easy to eat, taste good, and are high in nutrients. These recipes make it easy to make sure that people who have had a tracheostomy get the food they need to heal and stay healthy in the long run.

These recipes help you get better by using foods that are high in vitamins, minerals, and antioxidants, like butternut squash, avocado, spinach, and berries.

They also improve your general health and vitality. Whether eaten on their own or as part of a well-balanced meal plan, flavorful purees and mixed meals are a tasty and healthy way for people to start healing and getting healthy again after surgery.

CHAPTER 6

MEALS PACKED WITH PROTEINS TO HELP YOU GET STRONG AND RECOVERY

Meals Full of Protein to Get Strong and Recover:

For people who have had tracheostomy surgery, getting the right nutrition is very important for their healing. When you have surgery or other medical treatment, your body needs certain nutrients to heal, rebuild tissues, and get stronger. Protein stands out as one of these nutrients that is very important for helping muscles heal and recover generally. So, adding meals high in protein to the diet after surgery is very important for speeding up recovery and promoting long-term health. This complete guide to the best food after surgery includes protein-rich recipes designed to help with tracheostomy recovery. It includes meal plans, healing recipes, and expert tips for long-term health.

Many people love salmon because it is high in protein and omega-3 fatty acids, which help with healing after surgery. After all, they reduce inflammation. Grilling salmon keeps all of its health benefits and makes it taste better.

With its tangy lemon-dill sauce, this dish is a breath of fresh air, and the sauce makes the tender salmon even softer. The lemon dill sauce not only makes the food taste better, but it's also good for you because it contains vitamin C from the lemon and antioxidants from the dill. This high-protein meal not only helps muscles heal but also boosts the immune system, which speeds up the healing process after tracheostomy surgery.

Black bean and quinoa salad:

Quinoa is a great plant-based source of protein, which makes it a useful addition to the tracheostomy recovery diet, especially for people who like to eat veggie or vegan food. When you add black beans to this salad, it becomes a complete protein, which means it has all the important amino acids your body needs to grow and repair cells.

Also, quinoa has a lot of fiber, which helps digestion and keeps the gut healthy, which is very important during the recovery process. The different colored veggies and herbs in the salad not only make it taste better, but they also give you vitamins, minerals, and phytonutrients that are good for your health. People who are trying to get better can eat this hearty and healthy salad as an enjoyable meal.

Turkey meatballs in tomato sauce:

Turkey meatballs are a lean source of protein, which makes them perfect for people who want to cut back on fat while still getting enough protein while recovering from a tracheostomy. When paired with a tasty tomato sauce, these meatballs make a hearty and satisfying meal.

Also, turkey meat has a lot of nutrients, like zinc and B vitamins, which are very important for the nervous system and for using energy.

People can help their bodies recover while still eating a healthy, balanced diet by choosing lean protein sources like turkey. Adding these turkey meatballs in marinara sauce to your post-surgery meal plan is an easy and tasty way to get protein.

Tofu baked in a Teriyaki sauce:

Tofu is a flexible protein source that can help with tracheostomy healing. It is a mainstay of vegetarian and vegan diets. When you bake tofu with teriyaki glaze, the high protein content of the tofu and the savory sweetness of the teriyaki sauce work together to make a tasty and filling dish.

Tofu also has a lot of iron and calcium, which are important minerals for health and healing.

The teriyaki sauce gives the tofu more flavour and moisture, which makes it a good choice for people whose taste buds have changed after surgery.

By adding baked tofu with teriyaki glaze to the meal plan, people can enjoy a protein-rich dish that helps them heal and stay healthy in the long run while they are recovering from a tracheostomy.

 meals that are high in protein are very important for helping with strength and healing during tracheostomy rehabilitation. The above recipes offer healthy and tasty choices that can be changed to fit the dietary needs of people who have recently had surgery. People can speed up their recovery and improve their general health and vitality by adding these healing recipes to their meal plans along with expert tips for long-term wellness.

CHAPTER 7
DESSERTS AND TREATS THAT MAKE YOU FEEL GOOD

During the healing process after a tracheostomy, patients may have changes in their appetite and taste preferences due to things like medications, pain, or changed senses. Incorporating comforting treats and sweets into their diet can not only make them feel good but also help them meet their nutritional needs. The sweets on this list were chosen because they are easy on the throat, soothing, and full of healing nutrients.

Cookies with banana and muesli:

Cookies made with bananas and muesli are tasty treats that are both sweet and healthy. Not only are bananas high in potassium, which is good for your heart and muscles, but they also make the cookies soft and moist, which makes them easier for people with tracheostomy tubes to take.

On the other hand, muesli has a lot of fiber, which helps your body digest food and keep blood sugar levels steady. Putting these things together makes banana oatmeal cookies, a tasty dessert that you can enjoy without feeling bad.

Applesauce muffins are another comforting treat that can help people who have had tracheostomy surgery get better. Applesauce can be used instead of oil or butter in standard muffin recipes to make them sweeter and lower in fat while still adding flavour and moisture. Also, applesauce is easy to take and doesn't hurt the throat, so it's great for people who have tracheostomy tubes. You can change these muffins by adding things like nuts or spices for extra flavor and health benefits.

Creamy rice pudding is a traditional dessert that can help with tracheostomy healing by being comforting and healthy.

Rice pudding is made with cooked rice, milk, and sweeteners like honey or sugar. It has a creamy texture that is easy to swallow and feels good in your stomach. Because rice is a mild food that won't irritate the throat, it's good for people with sensitive throats. Milk also adds protein and calcium to the treat, which helps bones and muscles heal. By adding rice pudding to their diet, patients can enjoy a comforting treat that will also help them get better.

Mango coconut popsicles that are cold:

Mango coconut popsicles are a refreshing and tropical take on traditional desserts. They are a great treat for people who are healing from tracheostomy surgery. Not only are mangoes tasty, but they are also full of vitamins and antioxidants that help your body fight off disease and heal itself. Coconut milk has a creamy texture and a mild coconut flavor. It also has healthy fats that help your body absorb nutrients. Patients can enjoy a tasty snack that helps soothe their throats and gives them the nutrients they need to heal by mixing mangoes and coconut milk and freezing the mixture into popsicles.

 comforting desserts and treats are very important for helping people who have had tracheostomy surgery meet their nutritional needs and improve their general health. Patients can enjoy tasty treats that are easy on the throat and full of needed nutrients by adding these healing recipes to their diet. Planning meals and getting advice from experts can also speed up the healing process and make sure that the person stays healthy in the long run.

CHAPTER 8
ADVICE ON HOW TO PLAN AND CHANGE MEALS

Planning meals and making changes to your routine are important parts of getting better after tracheostomy surgery.

This complete guide aims to teach you how to plan meals well, change recipes to fit your specific dietary needs, and add variety and flavor to your diet for the best recovery after surgery.

Making Plans Ahead of Time to Save Time

During the time it takes to heal after tracheostomy surgery, ease is very important. Making food plans ahead of time can make things a lot easier for both the patient and the people who are caring for them.

Making a meal plan for the week makes sure that all of your meals contain the ingredients you need and takes the stress out of making meals every day.

To avoid getting too tired, it's best to plan meal prep sessions for when you're feeling your most energetic.

When planning meals, you might want to choose foods that are easy to make and don't require a lot of chewing or swallowing, since these things may be hard while you're recovering.

Kitchen tools like slow cookers, blenders, and food mixers can make preparing meals easier by streamlining the process. Making a lot of meals at once and saving them in single servings can also save time and effort on busy days.

Changing recipes to fit dietary needs

Tracheostomy patients often have special food needs because they can't swallow as well and need different nutrients.

Making changes to recipes to meet these needs is important for making sure people get the right nutrition and help them heal after surgery. Check out these changes:

• Texture Change: If a person has trouble eating, changing the texture of food can make it safer for them to eat.

Foods that are blended or pureed until they are smooth can be easier to swallow while still keeping their health benefits. People who have a tracheostomy should eat soft foods like soups, stews, mashed potatoes, and milkshakes.

• Nutrient-Rich Ingredients: Using nutrient-dense ingredients in cooking is very important for helping the body heal.

Focus on eating a range of fruits and vegetables along with lean proteins like chicken, fish, tofu, and legumes to get the vitamins and minerals your body needs. Eating whole carbs like oats, quinoa, and brown rice can also help keep your diet healthy.

• Adding more flavor: People who have had a tracheostomy may notice changes in their sense of smell and taste, which can make them less hungry and less interested in eating.

Try different herbs, spices, and seasonings to make food taste better and look better.

Aromatic herbs like rosemary, basil, and cilantro can give recipes more depth, and citrus fruits and vinegar-based dressings can add a tangy kick.

• Strategies for Staying Hydrated: Tracheostomy patients must stay properly hydrated to avoid problems like mucus buildup and thirst.

Besides drinking water, adding foods that are high in water, like cucumbers, watermelon, and soups with broth, to your meals can also help you get enough fluids.

Including Different Tastes and Offerings

Staying on a varied and tasty diet is important for long-term compliance with food guidelines and to avoid getting bored. For tracheostomy patients, meals can stay interesting and fun by using a range of products, flavors, and cooking methods.

Try out different types of food and cooking methods to make your diet more interesting. You might want to try Indian, Thai, or Mediterranean food, which are all known for using a lot of herbs, spices, and other fragrant ingredients. Adding colourful fruits and veggies to food not only makes it look better but also gives you a lot of different nutrients and antioxidants.

Involving the patient in planning and making decisions about meals also gives them the power to own their food choices and tastes. Get comments from people and change recipes to fit their tastes and needs.

Also, don't forget how important appearance is— arranging meals in a way that looks good can make them more appealing and fun to eat.

planning meals and making adjustments that work for each person are important parts of tracheostomy rehab because they make sure that patients get enough nutrition while also helping them heal and be healthy overall.

Tracheostomy patients can have a pleasant and healthy diet while they are recovering by planning for ease of preparation, changing recipes to fit dietary needs, and adding variety and flavor to meals.

CHAPTER 9
SUPPORT AND ENCOURAGEMENT FOR EMOTIONS

Emotional health is very important during the healing process after tracheostomy surgery. During physical rehabilitation, the mental side is often forgotten, but it is just as important for a full recovery. People who are having tracheostomy surgery may feel a lot of different feelings, from worry and fear to anger and sadness. To improve mental health and make the healing go more smoothly, it's important to recognize and deal with these feelings.

Why emotional health is important

It's impossible to say enough about how important mental health is during tracheostomy recovery. Patients who are still dealing with the effects of surgery may face a wide range of mental problems.

Having to depend on medical devices and making sudden changes to your lifestyle can make you feel vulnerable and unsure. Another thing that adds to the mental stress is not being able to talk clearly because of the tracheostomy tube. Ignoring these emotional effects can make it harder for the patient to heal and make the whole experience worse.

Sharing Food and Help to Get to Know Each Other

People have known for a long time that food is more than just something to eat. It can also bring people together and make them feel better.

When someone is recovering from a tracheostomy, making and sharing meals can be a powerful way to build social support. Family and friends can show they care by making healthy meals that are specifically designed to meet the patient's nutrition needs. Involving the patient in making meals as much as possible can also help them feel more normal and give them more power while they are recovering.

 Also, eating with others can be a way for people to talk about their feelings and connect, which can improve relationships and help people get through hard times.

Words have an amazing power to lift people and give them hope, especially when things are bad. Positive affirmations and words of support can make a huge difference for people who are going through the difficult process of tracheostomy recovery.

 The words and actions of loved ones, carers, and healthcare workers all play a big part in giving emotional support. Assuring the patient of your support, telling them stories of strength, and having faith in their ability to get through tough times can all be very simple but true actions that can help them heal emotionally. Also, supporting patients to do self-reflective activities like journaling or mindfulness meditation can help them deal with their feelings and find peace within themselves during the rough times of recovery. People who have tracheostomy surgery can handle the challenges of recovery with strength and resilience if they prioritize emotional support and encouragement. This will ultimately make the shift to long-term wellness easier.

CONCLUSION

Getting through the recovery process after surgery, especially if you had a tracheostomy, requires a thorough approach that includes both medical care and full nutritional support. This guide tries to be a complete resource for people going through the difficult process of recovery by giving them information about the importance of nutrition, useful tips on how to make meals, and a wide range of healing foods that are designed to help with the best possible recovery and long-term health.

We've talked about the importance of nutrient-dense soups and broths, soft, easy-to-swallow foods, flavorful purees and blended meals, protein-rich foods for strength and healing, and sweets and treats that make you feel good. Each recipe was carefully made to prioritize both nutrition and taste because enjoying and feeling good are important parts of the healing process.

In addition to talking about the physical parts of recovery, this book has also stressed how important it is to have emotional support and encouragement. Mind and body are linked, so we've stressed how important it is to take care of your emotions and build relationships through food and support.

As people start their recovery, the tips given for planning meals and making changes are very helpful for making sure that meals are realistic, varied, and meet dietary needs. People can improve their cooking experience while also helping their bodies heal by planning, making changes to recipes as needed, and using a variety of flavors.

This complete guide is a light of hope and strength for people who are going through the difficult process of recovering from surgery. By following the rules of nutrition, culinary creativity, and emotional strength, people can start a path to better health and vitality, giving them the tools and information, they need for long-term wellness.